THE
IRRITABILITY
CURE

*HOW TO STOP
BEING ANGRY,
ANXIOUS AND
FRUSTRATED
ALL THE TIME*

DOC ORMAN, M.D.

Published By:

TRO Productions, LLC
P.O. Box 768
Sparks, Maryland 21152

In association with TCK Publishing

www.TCKPublishing.com

DISCLAIMERS AND LEGAL NOTICES

Both the author and publisher of this book have strived to be as accurate and complete as possible in the creation of this information product. While all attempts have been made to verify the accuracy of the information contained herein, there is no warranty either expressly stated or implied of complete or permanent accuracy. After all, knowledge does evolve and change.

The author and publisher and any subsequent distributors of this work also assume no responsibility for any errors, assumptions, or interpretations you might make as result of consuming this information. You are solely responsible for how you choose to understand and make use of this information. Please use prudent judgment in attempting to apply any strategies, exercises, or other recommendations suggested herein. Also, any perceived slights of specific persons, peoples, or organizations are unintentional.

This book is also not intended to be a substitute or replacement for competent medical or psychological treatment when these may be needed. If you suffer from very severe anxiety, severe phobias, severe depression or any other serious mental health condition, the advice in the book may not be appropriate or sufficient for you. You are advised to consult and work with an experienced mental health professional, if you are not already doing so.

Also, if you believe that your symptoms or your problems are beginning to get worse as you read this book, you should stop reading it immediately and consult a trained health professional.

Dr. Mort Orman is a board-certified Internal Medicine physician. While he has been successfully helping and coaching people to overcome their stress and anxiety related problems for more than 30 years, he is not a licensed or practicing mental health professional. Therefore, you need to evaluate and personally assess all advice and suggestions put forth in this book in this light.

Bottom line: you are 100% responsible for how you interpret and make use of the information in this book. So please do so wisely.

CONTENTS

INTRODUCTION

My name is Mort (Doc) Orman, M.D. and want to welcome you to this short but powerful self-help guide on how to stop being irritable.

If you are a person who frequently gets irritated, you know how big a problem this can be. Little things that don't bother most other people set you off in ways that stir your emotions and rob you of your calmness and peace of mind.

Your relationships can suffer, you can lash out at people you care about, and your own sense of confidence and self-control can also be diminished.

It's not much fun to go through life feeling irritated most of the time. But as much as you might dislike this feeling, you've probably found it hard to stop. At least until now.

PURPOSE OF THIS GUIDE

The primary purpose of this guide is to teach you how to reduce or eliminate 75% or more of your irritability.

It will also show you how to stop getting irritated, anxious or frustrated by things that truly are insignificant.

Why haven't you already been able to succeed at getting rid of your irritability? The main reasons are:

> You don't understand your irritability problem correctly.

> You've never been taught to understand the causes of your irritability correctly.

> You haven't been given the best coping strategies.

> In short, you don't have a solid blueprint for making the changes you desire.

Your 5-Step Master Plan For Irritability

This brief but powerful guide is going to give you a **5-step master plan** for reducing and eventually eliminating your irritability. It's a plan that I have used to master my own irritability problem. And it's also the same plan I have taught to many others, who have found it to be helpful as well.

Here's a quick overview of the five main parts of this master plan:

1. **Identify** your irritability problem correctly.
2. Understand what you can and can't **change** about it.
3. **Discover** your present relationship to being irritated.
4. Identify the true **causes** of your problem.
5. **Learn** how to make your irritability quickly disappear.

I'll be covering each of these five steps in much more detail shortly. But first, let me tell you some things about who I am and why you might want to pay very close attention to what I am about to tell you.

MY OWN PERSONAL VICTORY OVER IRRITABILITY

I am a 65-year-old Internal Medicine physician, author, speaker, stress coach, and founder of The Stress Mastery Academy. For the past 30 years, I've been helping people eliminate many types of stress in their lives, with great success.

I have conducted hundreds of seminars and workshops on how to reduce stress for doctors, nurses, veterinarians, business executives, college students, medical students, psychologists, the clergy, and even the F.B.I.

I have written several popular books about stress, including several unique self-help guides similar to this one. I have also been the official sponsor of National Stress Awareness Month every April in the U.S. since 1992.

But for the first 30-plus years of my life, I was frequently plagued by high levels of stress, which I could never figure out how to handle. I was angry, frustrated, anxious, irritable, and unhappy much of the time. I had trouble maintaining long-term relationships with other people, and even though I managed to get through medical school and a three-year residency training program, I was not a happy camper, even though others viewed me as a successful and competent professional.

Inside, however, I was desperately searching for answers to my emotional and interpersonal problems, but none of the so-called 'solutions' I was able to find made much of a lasting difference.

Then, several years after I opened my medical practice, I had the good fortune to meet and study with some very enlightened teachers. Little by little, I began to understand why none of the traditional coping strategies I had tried were helping, and I began to get glimpses of new ways of thinking that eventually did help me change.

And the changes I was able to produce in my life wildly exceeded all my expectations. Not only that, but these changes have continued to last and benefit me for more than 30 years now!

I almost never get frustrated, anxious, or irritated anymore. I have been happily married to my wife Christina for 28 years, and even when I do become irritated every once in a while, I know exactly how to make this feeling quickly disappear whenever I want.

So, don't let the small number of pages in this guide make you think it couldn't be of much lasting value to you.

I've taken all the key lessons I have learned over the past 30 years about how to stop being irritable and have condensed them into five main steps that you can easily learn about in just a few pages.

Once you know about these five steps, along with the powerful principles they contain, you will have a fantastic **master plan** for reducing your irritability that you can benefit from for the rest of your life. And you can use the same basic plan for reducing anxiety, frustration, and other negative emotions, with just a few modifications.

Now, even though the master plan you're going to receive here is one of the best you will find anywhere, it is not a magical quick-fix solution. Even though you will gain many new insights from reading this guide, you are not going to wake up tomorrow morning and magically be free of your irritability.

Yes, you can eventually accomplish this goal, just like I did, but it's not going to happen overnight. The principles and strategies you're going to learn about in this guide require a good deal of practice and trial-and-error learning before you'll begin to see results.

But at least you will have a **solid game plan** that can help you achieve your goal.

I wish I had received this type of game plan when I was struggling to cope with my irritability many years ago. But none was around. I had to discover the secrets I'm going to teach you here the hard way. But thanks to this guide, you will now have a huge advantage that I didn't have.

So please pay close attention to each of the five steps in this master plan. Then go out and try to apply them in your life. I think you'll find that they work and that you can achieve a great deal of relief from them. Some of them may surprise you. Some may even shock you. But that's okay. Because if they help you, as I believe they will, you won't really care.

That's all I wanted to say for an introduction. Now, let's move on to step #1.

STEP 1

IRRITABILITY ISN'T YOUR PROBLEM... SOMETHING ELSE IS!

The first step to solving any problem in life is to **define your problem** correctly.

With regard to feeling irritable all the time, it's important to know that 'irritability' isn't really your problem. **Anger** is.

You see, 'irritability' is just a camouflage term invented to obscure what's really going on. Whenever we say we are feeling 'irritated', what's actually happening is we're getting angry over minor things—things that don't usually anger other people—and we are doing this way more frequently than we should.

Now you might be thinking that it doesn't make much difference whether you call your problem 'getting irritable all the time' or 'getting angry all the time'...but it does.

Irritability is not an easy problem to get your arms around. It's really a description of how your body is feeling—in a general sense—and therefore it's **not a well-defined problem** you can zero in on and aggressively attack.

Anger, on the other hand, is a very specific human emotion. There is nothing general, nebulous, or mysterious about it.

Anger has very specific causes, and when you know how to identify these causes, you can attack them with laser-focused precision and a very high degree of success.

In addition, calling your problem 'irritability' immediately throws you into a victim position. It makes you feel like you are constantly at the mercy of how your body is feeling and reacting at any point in time, and there's little you can do to control these.

On the other hand, the moment you say "I'm feeling irritated right now, **therefore I must be angry** about something" you are no longer a victim of how your body is behaving. You are now in position to deal with the source of your problem—getting angry—instead of the end result—feeling irritated and all the body sensations that go along with this.

I hope you can clearly see now that there is a HUGE difference in whether you think your problem is irritability or whether you know that it is really anger.

It's Nice To Think You Are Irritated

Here's another reason you should stop thinking your problem is 'irritability'. We often use this nicer-sounding term to delude both ourselves and others about how we REALLY feel.

Sometimes, it is hard for us to admit how really **pissed** we are. We don't like to see ourselves as angry, hostile people. And the angrier we feel inside, the more we want to tone it down and try to appear that we are not so strongly upset.

So we've invented this term called 'irritability' to soften the blow just a bit. It's kind of like the way politicians often invent nice sounding terms for new laws or programs that often have very sinister effects. Like the 'Affordable Care Act' that's going to end up costing trillions and trillions of dollars.

So stop pussy-footing around and pretending that you are a nice, caring, loving person most of the time. *The truth is that if you are frequently feeling irritated, you have a serious anger problem.* And while I'm sure you are a very nice and caring person, your anger problem—at a very basic level— is really not all that different from people who suffer from road rage or who respond to their angry feelings by acting violently towards others.

They have the same core anger problem that you have. The only difference is that you are caring and sensitive enough not to act out your feelings of anger. But the intensity of your upsets can sometimes be just as strong and just as frequent, and just as damaging to the quality of your life and to the quality of your relationships as it is for others who are more demonstrable with their angry feelings.

I know it may not be pleasant to think of yourself as having a serious anger problem, but trust me on this...you do. And the first step to overcoming this problem is to accept this truth about yourself and then commit to doing something about it.

Remember, anger can be attacked and defeated. Irritability cannot.

So making this subtle shift in how you define your problem is the first big step to ending your irritability issues...once and for all.

STEP 2

YOU CAN'T REALLY STOP BEING IRRITABLE

The next thing you need to understand is that if you've been suffering with irritability for any length of time, **you're not going to be able to stop being irritable.**

I know this may be shocking news, especially since the promise I made to you in the Introduction to this guide is that I'm going to show you how to stop being irritable much of the time. But in order to do this, I first have to inform you that you're not going to be able to stop.

Yes, I know this doesn't make much sense right now, but it's true nonetheless. Let me explain.

Why am I asking you to believe that one of the **key secrets** to stopping yourself from feeling irritable all the time is to accept the fact that you can't really stop?

How can these two seemingly contradictory statements both be true?

The answer is simple: it's because both are actually true...at the very same time.

In order to stop yourself from being irritable, one of the most important things you need to understand—right from the start—is that you can't stop yourself from being irritable...at least not in the short run.

Maybe way down the road...months or years from now, little things that set you off today may not set you off then. But for now, things that set you off today and make you feel irritated are going to continue to set you off tomorrow, and the next day, and the day after that, etc.

You've got to give up your dream of a magic miracle cure. You are going to continue to get irritated, once you complete reading this guide, just as frequently as you do today.

And I don't care how much you learn about this problem, from this guide or from anywhere else, or how many new insights you gain into why you become irritable so easily...*you're not going to magically stop this from happening.*

IRRITABILITY IS A BODY PROBLEM

The reason for this is that irritability is a **conditioned body response**. The reason why you are so irritable today is because your body has become conditioned, over time, to habitually respond in irritable ways.

You have habitually **looked at** things in certain ways, **thought about** things in certain ways, **perceived** things in certain ways, **felt about** things in certain ways, and **responded to** things in certain ways...that these now have become conditioned, automatic, irritability responses in your body. The tendency to become irritated has not just become ingrained in your mind, but in your physical being as well.

In other words, irritability has become part of the **physical structure of your body**...and this is why no matter how much you learn about it, it's not going to go away.

It's No Mystery Anymore

The reason why you become more easily irritated than others is because **your body** is different from theirs. You have simply practiced the ways of thinking, perceiving, and responding that produce irritability more often and more passionately than they have. And now this pattern of responding has become part of you (i.e. your body).

It now has a life of its own—becoming triggered **automatically** by certain events or circumstances that habitually set you off and make you instantly feel upset (i.e. angry).

So the second step in your master plan for coming to terms with your automatic, conditioned irritability is to realize that your body has become programmed to respond in exactly this way…time and time again…and you can't really stop it or control it.

Yes, you may be able to do things to hide your irritability, or suppress it, or mask it with alcohol, drugs, food, etc. You may even decide to express your irritability to others. But one thing you are not going to be able to do is stop it from happening in the first place. Your irritability is now like your body' **knee-jerk reflex**, or any other automatic body reaction, like becoming startled when you hear a loud noise, or feeling either embarrassed or proud when someone publically complements you.

IT'S PARADOXICAL

Yet, here I am telling you that you can't stop your automatic irritability, but you still can discover how to stop being irritable. Once again, how can these two seemingly contradictory statements both be true?

They are both true because they are statements made in two very different contexts.

Let me illustrate with an example. It's much like saying you can both win an argument in a relationship with someone and lose at the same time. When viewed from a similar context, both statements cannot be true at the same time. You cannot win and lose an argument at the very same time.

However, if you look at the second statement from a different—and broader—context, you can do both. You can win an argument in your relationship with someone you care about and lose something else with regard to the future of that relationship.

If the other person ends up resenting you for winning the argument, you may have 'won the battle but lost the war' in the process. So, when viewed from two very different (and valid) contexts, two seemingly contradictory statements can both end up being true at the very same time.

Let's now translate this to your irritability problem. In one context (i.e. how your body has become conditioned to respond over time), you can't stop yourself from automatically responding by becoming irritable over little things that might not bother other people.

But in a completely different context (i.e. **how you choose to relate to your irritability**, once it has become triggered within you), you can definitely choose to relate to your irritability differently, and this can be the key to learning how to quickly stop feeling irritated, once it has automatically become triggered within you.

But before you can change and improve the way you relate to your irritability (anger) once it gets triggered within you, first you have get clear about what your present relationship is to it.

This brings us to Step 3 in your master plan.

YOU NEED TO UNDERSTAND YOUR CURRENT RELATIONSHIP TO FEELING IRRITATED

Here's another very important piece of the puzzle.

Not only do you automatically respond to certain things and events in your life with irritability, but you also have an **automatic relationship** to your irritability once it appears within your body. In other words, you have an automatic way of relating to your irritability that you probably haven't examined very critically.

What this guide and master plan is really all about is helping you realize that while you may not have much choice or control over whether and when you get irritated, you do have a tremendous amount of personal control over how you are going to relate to feeling irritated, whenever this occurs for you.

This is where you can step in and do something to stop yourself from feeling irritated (i.e. being angry)—not by preventing it from occurring in the first place—but by learning how to make it go away very quickly, once it has become triggered within you.

You absolutely do have this **awesome power**—to quickly reduce or eliminate your irritability anytime it occurs—but in order to access this power, you'll have to shift the type of relationship you automatically tend to have towards it.

WHAT IS YOUR AUTOMATIC RELATIONSHIP TO BECOMING IRRITATED?

What can we say about your present, automatic relationship to becoming irritated?

Basically, it can be described as looking for ways to suppress your irritability, hide the fact that you are feeling irritated (angry), or express your feelings of anger by letting others around you know how irritated they have made you feel.

Thus, whenever your body becomes triggered to feel irritated, you have some variation of automatically relating to this feeling by either going with the irritability or fighting against it. *In either case, your relationship is fundamentally built upon the presupposition that you are justified in feeling irritable, and that therefore the underlying thoughts, assumptions, and perceptions which are creating your feeling state are accurate and correct.*

In other words, your present relationship to becoming angry and feeling irritated is to *automatically assume that you have very good grounds for feeling irritated*, and that the only issue remaining is to decide whether to suppress or express how you feel.

With this type of automatic way of relating to your irritability, it will rarely occur to you that you may not actually have good grounds for feeling irritated in the first place, since your automatic way of relating is to assume just the opposite.

This is exactly the same relationship to getting angry that people who suffer from road rage have. It is also how people who repeatedly engage in verbal or physical abusive behaviors automatically relate to their internal feelings of anger.

It's also the same basic automatic relationship to becoming angry that most people have, so if you want to eventually become free of your irritability, *you are going to have to consciously choose to adopt a very different relationship to it.*

This is the 'secret sauce' to knowing how to make your irritability lessen and quickly disappear. *It's all about the type of relationship you choose to have towards your feelings of irritability and anger, once they occur for you.*

In the final two steps of your 5-step master plan, I will show you what type of relationship works better than the automatic one you presently have. I will also show you how you can benefit greatly from adopting this new type of relationship, not just in reducing your feelings of irritability, but in reducing your anxiety, your frustrations, and improving many other areas of your life as well.

But before you can even begin to think about how you are going to create a new and more rewarding relationship toward your irritability, you first have to understand the true **causes of anger** in any human being. The chances are good that you've probably been badly misinformed about these causes for most of your life.

Thus, it's no accident you haven't been able to solve your irritability problem in the past, no matter how hard you may have tried. This is because you haven't been focused on the right set of causes.

Hopefully, this is another huge benefit you will gain from this guide. And once you do understand these causes more clearly, I think it will help you to better deal with anger of all types in your life, as well as giving you much more insight and empathy for why other people get angry as well.

After all, we are all human beings, and as you are about to discover, we all get angry for exactly the same reasons and causes.

STEP 4

YOU NEED TO BE CLEAR ABOUT UNDERLYING CAUSES

Before diving right into this very important subject, let's take a moment to review what you've learned so far.

In Step 1 of your master plan, we clarified that irritability is not really your problem. Rather it is frequently getting angry over minor or trivial things that don't usually bother most other people.

Then, in Step 2, I pointed out that frequently getting angry over minor, trivial things is a **body problem** and therefore is not something you can hope to directly change or control.

As I am sure you already know, getting irritated frequently over very minor things is not something you actively choose to do. It is also not something you even want to do or like that you do. It just happens automatically for you now, and there's little you can do to stop or prevent this from continually happening over and over again.

In Step 3, I showed you that there is a way out of this seemingly hopeless condition. The way out is by first recognizing the type of **automatic relationship** you presently have to becoming irritated (angry), so you can begin to understand its weaknesses and design a new type of relationship that serves you much better in your life.

In order to do these two things—understand what's not so great about your present relationship to becoming angry all the time and then design a new and better relationship that overcomes the major deficiencies of your existing one—you first have to understand why the emotion of anger occurs for any human being, which obviously includes you as well.

So what exactly do you need to know in order to correctly understand the fundamental causes of anger in all human beings?

INTERNAL VS. EXTERNAL CAUSES

When it comes to recognizing the causes of our emotions, we are good at identifying certain types of causes and not very good at identifying others.

Consider the following example of John, a 35 year old sales executive, who frequently gets irritated (angry) when he gets stuck in a traffic jam:

John: *"I have a terrible time coping with traffic jams. I've got a very busy schedule, and I really get steamed when some jerk doesn't keep his eye on the road and causes me to miss an important meeting. Sure, I know what's causing my anger to occur, but most of the time, it's beyond my control."*

John thinks he correctly understands the causes of his automatic reactions of anger and irritability: **poor drivers**. But he's only identifying half the puzzle pieces.

Poor drivers are just part of the reason John gets so upset by traffic jams. There are other causes involved, but John doesn't recognize these causes, because they're not obvious to him.

If John did have all the puzzle pieces (causes) available to him, however, he would better understand why he gets so 'irritated' by traffic jams. He might even find that he has much more control over his reactions than he gives himself credit for.

OBVIOUS VS. HIDDEN CAUSES

All human emotions have two types of causes:

> ➢ Obvious Causes
> ➢ Hidden Causes

Obvious causes are the ones everyone usually notices. **Hidden causes** are the missing puzzle pieces most of us typically fail to recognize.

Look at the following list of obvious causes of stress in general for most human beings and note any that may have occurred for you in your life:

> ➢ Traffic jams
> ➢ Making a speech to a group
> ➢ Having a tight deadline to meet
> ➢ Having too many duties or responsibilities to fulfill
> ➢ Dealing with difficult people
> ➢ Conflicts with parents or relatives
> ➢ Losing your job or being worried about losing your job
> ➢ Dealing with illness or injury
> ➢ Dealing with illness or injury in a loved one
> ➢ Financial pressures
> ➢ Kids misbehaving or having problems

Now, how much of a role do you think these obvious causes played in your stress?

90% or more?

50%?

10% or less?

If you answered 90% or more, you probably have lots of company. This is how most of us, since early childhood, have been taught to think about the causes of our problems.

If you answered either 50% or 10%, you are much closer to the truth.

While obvious causes usually do play some role, the hidden causes of stress are either equally important or sometimes even more so.

So what are these hidden causes? And where do they come from?

The hidden causes of our emotions (and many other types of stress) are the **internal** thoughts, ideas, perceptions, and behaviors that exist **within us**, and which therefore are neither external to us nor are they usually as obvious.

These are the hidden, internal causes of our emotions, or missing puzzle pieces, that we often fail to recognize.

But once you know how to recognize these internal causes and have all the important causes of your anger—both obvious and hidden—in front of you, you will immediately see many more options for dealing with your anger problems than if you're only working with just the obvious causes.

HOW DO INTERNAL CAUSES CONTRIBUTE TO OUR GETTING ANGRY?

Let's return to John and his traffic jam problem.

What John didn't realize was that in addition to the obvious, external traffic jam, getting stuck in traffic also triggered certain internal thoughts, beliefs, and assumptions within him.

His attention was so focused, however, on just the obvious, external causes, that he never paid any attention to these internal patterns that were also contributing to his anger and irritability.

Take a look at the following list of **internal thoughts** that typically get triggered for most people when they unexpectedly find themselves delayed by a traffic jam.

Notice if any of these internal thoughts have ever occurred for you, under similar circumstances:

INTERNAL THOUGHTS COMMONLY TRIGGERED BY TRAFFIC JAMS

"This shouldn't be happening to me."

"Terrible things will happen if I don't get to my destination on time."

"I should always be able to go where I want, whenever I want."

"Whoever caused this mess to occur must have been an imbecile."

"Somebody should have warned me about this tie up."

"Sitting in a traffic jam is a stupid waste of my time."

These usually unconscious, or sometimes semi-conscious, internal thoughts can add extra layers of anger and emotional distress to an already bothersome situation.

John believed his traffic jam stress was caused primarily by other motorists. He never considered that his own internal thoughts might also be playing an even bigger role.

KEY PRINCIPLE:

It is rarely external events or the behavior of other people **alone** that cause us to get emotionally upset. Rather, it is the combination of external events, along with our own internal thoughts, beliefs, assumptions, perceptions, and behaviors, that together cause our emotions to occur.

WHAT ROLE DO OUR HABITUAL ACTIONS AND BEHAVIORS PLAY?

Let's examine some typical action patterns that might also contribute to traffic jam anger. Notice if any of the following actions (or lack of acting) have ever caused you to end up stuck in a traffic jam:

- ➤ Failing to listen to traffic reports or check for delays before venturing out.

- ➤ Choosing a route that's quicker and more direct, but leaves you fewer escape options if traffic should come to a halt.

- ➤ Blaming yourself for being "stupid" enough to get stuck.

> Leaving only enough time for your journey if everything goes smoothly, but no extra time to allow for unexpected problems.

> Complaining and getting more and more angry and upset, instead of creatively finding something of value to do while you are waiting.

Each of these action patterns frequently plays a role in contributing to any traffic jam anger or irritation people experience.

NOTE: This way of thinking about anger and other human emotions is consistent with similar approaches advocated by leading cognitive and behavioral psychologists.

HOW TO IDENTIFY THE HIDDEN, INTERNAL CAUSES OF HUMAN ANGER

In this next part of your guide and master plan, I'm going to teach you how to easily recognize the internal causes of anger, whenever you are feeling irritated or otherwise experiencing this very common human emotion.

The reason this type of knowledge is so important is because once you know how to pinpoint both the obvious and hidden causes of anger or irritation, you will then be in position to make these feelings quickly disappear....whenever you want....without needing to use cigarettes, alcohol, drugs, food, relaxation, physical exercise, or any type of stress management technique.

NOTE: While I will focus only on the specific emotion of ANGER in this guide, the general principles for identifying the hidden, internal causes of this emotion apply to all other emotions we commonly experience, such as anxiety, guilt, sadness, and frustration. This is because the ability to master any stressful problem in life boils down to how good you are at **two key skills**:

1) The ability to specifically pinpoint all of the major causes of the problem—including hidden, internal causes which are not always in clear view;

2) The ability to know what to do about those causes, especially the internal ones, once you correctly identify them.

TRIGGERS AND CAUSES

Human emotions have both **triggers** and **causes**:

Triggers are **events** (usually external to us) that **activate** causes.

Causes (always within us) determine which specific **emotion** occurs.

Causes are the specific internal thoughts and action patterns within us. For example, say that a friend steals money from you one day, and when you become aware of this you become enraged. The fact that your friend stole from you was the external, obvious event that **triggered** your emotion. The fact that you became angry (enraged) as a result of this trigger means that certain very specific anger-producing thoughts and actions patterns must have become activated within you.

INVISIBLE, INTERNAL CAUSES

Imagine that you're sitting in front of a desktop computer. You've just pressed the letter "A" key on your keyboard, and the letter "A" immediately appears on your monitor screen.

What caused this outcome to occur? Pressing the "A" key, right?

Not exactly. Pressing the "A" key was just the triggering event.

A **software program** also had to be running in the background of the computer.

Even though the software program isn't visible to you, it has to be there. Otherwise, the letter "A" would never have appeared on your monitor screen.

HUMAN EMOTIONS HAVE INVISIBLE CAUSES TOO

When events trigger emotions within us, there's always a very specific emotion-causing "program" running in the background (i.e. in our bodies). Unfortunately, we have not been taught to understand our emotions in this way.

Even worse, we've been repeatedly taught to believe that external events themselves directly cause our emotions to occur. This, in my opinion, is a gigantic failing of our educational system.

SPECIFIC EMOTIONS ALWAYS HAVE SPECIFIC CAUSES

The interesting thing about the internal causes of human emotions is they are exactly the same for all human beings.

For example, the specific internal thought patterns and action patterns that cause anger to occur for you...is exactly the same invisible "program" that causes anger to occur for human beings all over the globe.

This means that if someone in China becomes angry, and another person in Africa becomes angry, both are thinking and perceiving (at a very basic level) in exactly the same ways as you are thinking whenever you are feeling angry or irritated.

And if someone in America gets angry, regardless of the external triggering event, the same set of internal thoughts and action patterns must have been triggered within them as well.

The beauty of thinking about human emotions in this way is that once you learn to recognize the hidden internal causes that produce anger in one human being, you will at the very same time understand what causes anger to occur for all human beings.

> *Even more important, every time you become angry yourself, you'll immediately know the specific ways you must be thinking, perceiving, and acting in order for you to be experiencing this particular emotion (and not other ones).*

This is incredibly useful to know if you want to successfully deal with your anger, irritability, or any other emotion.

A NEW MODEL FOR UNDERSTANDING HUMAN EMOTIONS

Here's a simple model that can help you better visualize how human emotions occur:

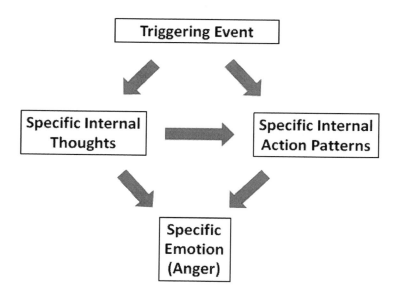

Both the triggering event and the emotion you feel are the **obvious** components of your experience.

However, if these are the only puzzle pieces you notice, you can't truly understand what's causing you to feel the way you do. But when you also learn to recognize the hidden, internal causes of your emotions, you then get a more complete picture of what is really going on.

THE INDEX CARD TECHNIQUE

I am now going to introduce you to a very powerful tool for recognizing the hidden causes of your emotions. I call this tool **The Index Card Technique**, and I have taught thousands of people how to use it, and benefit from it, during the past 30 years.

Here's how it works:

1. Identify the hidden, internal thoughts and action patterns responsible for any particular emotion.
2. Write these internal causes down on an index card.
3. Carry the card with you, or keep it handy.
4. Whenever you experience that emotion, take out your card and review its contents.

Whenever you are feeling that particular emotion, assume the thoughts and action patterns written on your card must have been triggered within you, whether you are consciously aware of them or not. Obviously, it might not always be practical to whip out your index card the moment you feel a strong emotion. But try using it to review things later on, once you've settled down and are away from the immediate situation.

THESE INDEX CARDS WON'T ELIMINATE YOUR EMOTIONS

It's important to understand, right from the start, that the Index Card Technique is only designed to help you **recognize** the hidden causes of your emotions. It is not a technique for getting rid of your unwanted emotions.

With regard to dealing with your feelings of irritability, I'll give you some tips for how to benefit from using your Anger Index Card in Step 5 of your master plan.

BUILDING YOUR CARD FOR ANGER (PART 1)

Let's now begin to build your index card for ANGER.

Anger-Producing Thoughts

Here are four ideas, assumptions, or thought patterns that must be present, in the background of your thinking/perceiving, in order for the emotion of anger or irritability to occur:

1. Someone did something they shouldn't have done.

2. Someone was hurt, harmed, humiliated, embarrassed, offended, disappointed, or otherwise inconvenienced by what was done.

3. Some person or persons (other than myself) were unilaterally responsible (i.e. to blame) for #1 and #2.

4. The offending person or persons should acknowledge what they did wrong, offer to make amends, and/or be punished.

NOTE: For thought pattern #1 above, you could also be angry at yourself, or at a pet, or at any other living creature, or even at an inanimate object, such as your car, your computer, or the hammer that somehow just struck your finger. If this is the case, simply adjust the above thought patterns accordingly.

Let's now look at each of these thought patterns in more detail.

Thought Pattern 1: Someone Did Something They Shouldn't Have Done

Whenever we feel angry, we've automatically assumed that someone did something **bad** or **wrong**—i.e., something they shouldn't have done.

Example: Consider our earlier example of a friend stealing money from us. When we found out about this, we immediately became angry. Why did we get angry?

Answer:

Puzzle piece #1—Our friend stole money from us (obvious cause or triggering event).

Puzzle piece #2—We automatically judged this behavior to be bad or wrong (hidden internal cause).

Thought Pattern 2: Someone Was Hurt, Harmed, Etc., By What Was Done

Whenever we feel angry, we also believe that someone (ourselves or others) was hurt, harmed, humiliated, embarrassed, offended, disappointed, or otherwise inconvenienced by what was done.

In other words, we must perceive (or imagine) that some major **negative impact** directly resulted from the bad or wrong behavior.

If we believe little or no harm or negative impact occurred, we don't usually get angry, even if someone did something they shouldn't have done.

Example: You're in a grocery store one day, and you witness a mother shopping with her young child. The child makes a fuss, and the mother angrily reacts by slapping the child very hard. You immediately feel angry. Once again, why did this specific emotion occur for you?

Answer:

Puzzle piece #1
The mother hit her child very hard for some trivial misbehavior (obvious cause or triggering event)

Puzzle piece #2
You automatically judged the mother's behavior to be bad or wrong (hidden internal cause).

Puzzle piece #3
You also automatically concluded that the child suffered hurt or harm—hurt in the immediate sense of physical pain, and possible harm in the longer sense due to potential psychological damage, especially if this mother's behavior continues, as it might (second hidden internal cause).

Let's now look at this same example from the mother's perspective, and see if we can understand (not necessarily forgive or condone) why she got so angry with her child.

Why did the mother become angry in this example?

Answer (Mother's Anger):

Puzzle piece #1
The child became very fussy (obvious cause or triggering event).

Puzzle piece #2
The mother judged her child's behavior to be very bad or wrong.

Puzzle piece #3
The mother judged that she was being negatively impacted as a direct result of the child's "misbehavior."

Note: We can't know for sure the exact thoughts or perceptions going on in the mind of another person. But we can be sure that if a person becomes clearly angry, some perception of immediate or future negative impact must have occurred. Also notice that the hidden causes of our own anger, from just witnessing such an event, are exactly the same hidden causes that provoked the mother to become angry at her child.

WHY PEOPLE HAVE DIFFERENT EMOTIONAL REACTIONS TO THE SAME EVENT

If you understand the first two anger-producing thought patterns above, you should be able to appreciate now why different people can have vastly different emotional reactions to the very same event.

It all has to do with the internal judgments, evaluations, and perceptions that get triggered within each individual.

1491 EXAMPLE

If you were alive in 1491 and you observed a boat with people on it disappear over the horizon, you would likely be overcome by strong feelings of sadness, grief, and horror.

Why? Because the prevailing thought patterns at that time were "the world is flat" and "if you go over the edge, you will certainly die." In 1491, those would have been the likely ideas triggered within your body by witnessing such an event.

Today, we see boats disappear over the horizon all the time, yet no strong emotions get triggered within us. Why? Because the prevailing thought patterns in our times are that "the world is round" and that disappearing over the horizon simply means you just "disappeared from view."

In this example, the same identical event, witnessed by two very different hypothetical people, living centuries apart, produced two completely different automatic emotional responses.

> *This also explains why you may become irritated very easily by minor or trivial events that don't seem to bother other people.*

The reason for this is that these minor events trigger anger-producing thought patterns within you, whereas they don't trigger the same thoughts and assumptions in others.

Thought Pattern 3: Someone Was Unilaterally to Blame

Simply judging something to be bad or wrong, and to have produced hurt, harm, or other negative impact, are not enough, by themselves, to produce the emotion of anger.

We also need to identify the responsible agent. This is required because we need to know where to direct our anger. In other words, we need to know who or what to be angry about (i.e., to blame).

UNILATERAL BLAME

We've been culturally conditioned to view **blame** from an Either/Or perspective. This means we tend to look for a primary agent to assign most or all of the blame to, while all other participants or factors are judged to be innocent.

This type of internal thought pattern is called **unilateral blame**, since it tends to be almost exclusively one-sided.

ANGER AND BLAME

Whenever we perceive something bad or wrong that results in hurt or harm, we will automatically seek to assign blame.

Examples: Take the two examples we've already considered.

A. In the first example (friend stealing money from us), our friend is perceived to be unilaterally to blame for his or her actions. After all, we didn't have anything to do with this person deciding to steal money from us.

B. In the second example, the mother was clearly to blame for hitting her child.

Even though we clearly observed that the child's behavior also played a role, we still tend to place the majority of blame on the mother.

THREE PRIMARY ANGER-PRODUCING THOUGHT PATTERNS

These first three thought patterns, which we have just discussed, are the **primary thought patterns** that cause anger to occur in human beings.

If any event triggers all three of these internal thought patterns within us, the emotion of anger will surely follow. On the other hand, if only one or two of these thought patterns get triggered (but not all three), it is unlikely that feelings of anger or irritation will occur.

Thought Pattern 4: The Offenders Should Acknowledge What They Did Wrong, Offer to Make Amends, and/or Be Punished

The fourth thought pattern is not a primary anger-producing requirement. It's a "bonus" thought pattern that is prevalent in our society and that intensifies our anger in most situations.

Example: Have you ever noticed what happens when someone does something bad or wrong that caused hurt or harm to another, and the person was clearly to blame for their actions, and then, when confronted, that person refuses to admit it?

Your anger gets worse, doesn't it?

This happens because we live in a society where our expectation is that people should acknowledge what they did wrong, especially when their wrongdoings negatively impacted others. We also expect them to make amends and/or be punished for their behavior.

When these social expectations are not fulfilled, our anger becomes intensified. Why? For exactly the same reasons our anger occurs in the first place. After all, if we expect a person to admit their wrongdoings and they refuse to comply, isn't this just another instance of them doing something bad or wrong? And isn't that person totally to blame for their refusal? And might we be disappointed, offended, or otherwise negatively impacted? Thus, this 4th thought pattern is just a repeat of the first three primary anger-producing thought patterns. Therefore, it follows very logically that our feeling of anger will intensify.

NOTE: While the internal "program" that produces anger in human beings is exactly the same for all of us, there is great variability in the external events that trigger these internal thought patterns. There is also variability in how emotions such as anger and irritability are felt and expressed by different people. For example, people have different standards for judging behaviors or events as being bad or wrong. Also, some people are highly in touch with their emotions, while others may suppress feelings of anger, or not feel much at all, even when they have been triggered to become angry inside (as measured and confirmed physiologically).

THE FRONT SIDE OF YOUR ANGER CARD

You now know the 3 primary and 1 bonus thought patterns that cause anger to occur for all human beings. This means you are now ready to create the front side of your Anger Index Card.

BUILDING YOUR ANGER INDEX CARD

Print out this page (if you can) and then cut out the information below and tape it or paste it onto a 3x5 index card. Alternatively, you could handwrite the information on a blank index card.

ANGER THOUGHT PATTERNS

1. Someone did something they shouldn't have done.

2. Someone was hurt, harmed, humiliated, embarrassed, offended, disappointed, or otherwise inconvenienced by what was done.

3. Some person or persons (other than myself) were unilaterally responsible (i.e. to blame) for #1 and #2.

4. The offending person or persons should acknowledge what they did wrong, offer to make amends, and/or be punished.

Congratulations! You are now halfway done creating your Anger Index Card.

In a few moments, we'll fill in the back side of the card (Action Patterns).

In Step 5 of your master plan, I'll show you how to make use of this index card, along with other strategies I'll also reveal to help you make your anger and irritability quickly and easily disappear whenever you want.

ANGER-PRODUCING ACTION PATTERNS

Here are the internal action patterns that either cause anger to occur for us or keep it from resolving quickly:

A. Failing to recognize how your own judgments, evaluations, and standards might not be valid for other people.

B. Failing to recognize how your own actions, past and present, may have contributed to what happened.

C. Justifying your anger, instead of looking within yourself for its internal causes.

D. Retaliating or seeking revenge, instead of openly and honestly dealing with what happened.

Anger-producing thought patterns and action patterns can mutually reinforce one another. So sometimes, action patterns may play a role in causing our emotions to occur. In general, however, thought patterns are more involved in the generation of our emotions, whereas action patterns often kick in later, either to intensify the emotion or keep it from quickly resolving.

Let's now examine each of the anger-producing action patterns listed above in more detail.

A) Failing to recognize how your own judgments, evaluations, and standards might not be valid for other people.

Often, we will judge other people's behaviors to be bad or wrong, based on our own personal standards, without being aware we are doing so. This gives us the illusion that whatever happened "really was bad" or "really was wrong," instead of the event being one thing and our internal judgments being quite another.

On the other hand, when you consciously remind yourself that what other people do—and your judgments about their actions—are **two different things**, the next logical question becomes "On what basis did I arrive at my conclusion?"

Often, the honest answer is you referenced **your own personal standards** for how you expect or believe people should behave. When you look at it in this way, the other person may not have done anything that was truly wrong!

Much of this internal judging activity goes on automatically, beyond our conscious awareness. This means we are usually unaware that:

We are actively judging other's behaviors to be bad or wrong.

We are doing so based on personal standards that may not be valid for others.

ARE OUR PERSONAL STANDARDS TRULY VALID FOR OTHERS?

When you get irritated with another person's behavior, was what that person did inherently bad or wrong? Or was it just different from how you would do things?

Ask yourself this question a few times, and you may begin to see just how misguided your automatic judgments frequently are.

B) Failing to recognize how your own actions, past and present, may have contributed to what happened.

This action pattern is related to our automatic assumptions of unilateral blame. This type of Either/Or thinking about blame frequently results in incorrect perceptions about what really happened.

When we automatically view other people as being unilaterally to blame, we often fail to recognize how our own actions, past and present, might have contributed to what happened.

Example: A friend starts acting mean and nasty towards you for no apparent reason.

You judge this behavior to be bad and wrong and begin to feel angry. You also judge your friend to be unilaterally to blame for behaving inappropriately.

But what if you did something days earlier that offended your friend?

Perhaps you didn't realize your friend felt offended by something you did or didn't do. So while it may have initially appeared that you were completely innocent in the matter, the truth may be otherwise.

C) Justifying your anger instead of looking within yourself for its internal causes.

As a result of doing seminars for thousands of individuals, I have occasionally met people who are highly attached to their anger and irritability.

These people are very quick to **justify their anger** as well as the "validity" of their personal evaluations and perceptions that fuel it. Such individuals find it very difficult to accept their own internal role in causing their anger to occur. They also feel threatened by anything that might lessen their anger or cast doubt on the importance they have assigned to this and other emotions.

If you tend to be a person who justifies your anger, and if you share similar concerns, please be reassured. Nothing in this guide or master plan will take away any of your emotions from you.

On the other hand, if you want to get rid of any negative emotions, such as frequent anger or irritability over minor or trivial things, this guide will give you insights and tools that may very well enable you to do this... but only when you choose to do so.

D) Retaliating or seeking revenge, instead of openly and honestly dealing with what happened.

Another very common action pattern that keeps anger from resolving is retaliating or seeking revenge. This is tied to the 4th anger-producing thought pattern we examined earlier.

When we perceive others to have done something bad or wrong, and they don't own up to it, we may want to punish them, or otherwise seek revenge.

To the other person, however, our retaliation seems like something bad and wrong that we are doing. So they get triggered to punish us in return. This vicious circle can go on for some time, until one or other party ceases to participate.

NOTE: It's also interesting to notice that while we are busy seeking revenge, we are also engaged in justifying our anger and failing to look at how our own actions (or misperceptions) might have contributed to what happened. Thus, we can be guilty of engaging in several anger-producing or anger-maintaining action patterns at the very same time.

TIP: Rent the movie "Tin Men" starring Richard Dreyfus and Danny DeVito. Set in Baltimore in the 1960's, this story is about two strangers, both of whom happen to be aluminum siding salesmen, who collide one day in a minor car accident.

As you watch this humorous tale of wildly escalating revenge-seeking behavior, notice how the entire script for this movie was taken straight from the thought patterns and action patterns that we just reviewed.

COMPLETING YOUR ANGER INDEX CARD

You are now ready to complete your Anger Index Card.

When you add the anger-producing Action Patterns to the back of your card, your index card will be complete.

Print out this page (again, if you can) and then cut out the information below and tape it or paste it to the back of your 3x5 Anger Index Card. Alternatively, you could handwrite the information on a blank index card.

ANGER ACTION PATTERNS

1. Failing to recognize how your own judgments, evaluations, and standards might not be valid for other people.

2. Failing to recognize how your own actions, past and present, may have contributed to what happened.

3. Justifying your anger, instead of looking within yourself for its internal causes.

4. Retaliating or seeking revenge, instead of openly and honestly dealing with what happened.

Congratulations! You have now completed your Anger Index Card.

THIS CARD WORKS....EVERY TIME!

Remember, if you're feeling angry at any time, or for any reason, you must be thinking and often behaving in exactly the ways listed on your Anger Index Card.

I have personally tested this Anger Index Card thousands of times, both in my own life and in my work with other people. And I have never found it to fail.

For example, whenever I am feeling angry, it always turns out that I am automatically thinking, perceiving, and often behaving in precisely the ways listed on this Anger Index Card. It doesn't matter whether I am consciously aware of having these internal thoughts, or of possibly behaving in these anger-generating ways.

When I use my index card to probe my inner thoughts and behaviors more deeply, I always find that I am guilty of automatically thinking and behaving in exactly these ways. No exceptions! Ever!

Your Irritability Should No Longer Be A Mystery To You

You now have a **fool-proof way** to always identify the hidden internal causes of anger or irritability anytime these feelings occur for you.

Thus, it should never again be a mystery to you why you get irritated in any situation.

While you may have previously thought it was the behavior of others, or the events that happen outside of you that cause you to become irritated, you can no longer afford to engage in this fantasy.

It's not the external events or behaviors of others that are causing you to feel irritated. Rather it is your own internal thought patterns and action patterns, which over the years have become programmed to occur in your body.

Now, however, you have a very simple tool—your Anger Index Card—to always know for sure exactly why you get irritated about anything!

Mystery resolved! Now, the only question remaining is what are you going to do with this knowledge? How can you use this new information to have much less anger and irritability in your life?

This question ultimately gets back to the type of relationship you adopt whenever you do become irritated.

By virtue of understanding the hidden internal causes of your anger, you are now in excellent position to create a new and much more powerful relationship to your automatic irritability problem, and to the automatic thought patterns and action patterns that get triggered within you to cause it to happen, over and over again.

HOW TO CREATE A NEW RELATIONSHIP TO YOUR IRRITABILITY THAT CAN ENABLE YOU TO MAKE IT QUICKLY DISAPPEAR WHENEVER YOU WANT!

O kay. It's now time to show you how to get some amazing results.

As with any high-quality self-help tool or master plan, I can show you what to do to reduce or eliminate a problem in your life, but I can't do the actual work for you.

Only you can take the information and guidance someone offers you and make the needed efforts to apply it correctly. If you do this with this guide, hopefully you'll be able to make the type of meaningful changes you desire, and that you were searching for when you originally became attracted to it.

With regard to changing yourself from a person who frequently becomes irritated over minor things into a person who hardly ever becomes irritated over anything, and who also knows how to quickly put an end to any unwanted feelings of anger or irritability, this is entirely possible for you to accomplish. But remember, it won't come easily, and it's definitely not going to happen overnight.

So far, I've given you four critically important steps to follow in an overall master plan for making this type of massive personal change. But all four of these steps taken together won't make any difference at all, if you fail to master this final game-changing step.

YOU'VE COME A LONG WAY...SO FAR

By reading this far in this guide, you've actually come quite a long way toward being able to finally solve your recurring irritability problem.

Here's what we've established so far:

You don't really have a problem with irritability—you are a person (probably a very good and kind person) who automatically gets angry over little things in life that don't really bother most other people.

You haven't been able to solve this recurring problem so far, mainly because you haven't understood that you can't really stop your body from getting irritated (at least not in the short run) and because you've never been taught to understand the true causes of anger correctly.

You've lived your life, so far, focusing mainly on external situations and events, including the external behaviors of other people around you, as the primary culprits for why you get so irritated. There's no need to feel bad about this, because almost everyone around you is doing the same thing as well.

However, you now have a clear understanding of the internal causes of anger and irritability, not just in yourself, but in all human beings as well.

You also now understand that you have an automatic relationship to your episodes of irritability, each time they occur for you, and this automatic relationship also extends to the thought patterns and action patterns that get triggered within you, and which drive your irritability to arise in the first place.

Prior to reading this guide, you could be forgiven because you may have had no idea what these hidden, internal anger-producing thought patterns and action patterns were. But now, you no longer have any excuses!

In short, you now know exactly what is causing your recurring feelings of irritability and how you are presently relating to them (I'll go over this relationship part again shortly).

The only question remaining is this: "what are you going to do now?" Are you going to continue going along with you old, automatic relationship to your recurring irritability (and the automatic thoughts and behaviors underlying it), or are you going to be open to learning how to create a new type of relationship that will serve you much better…for the rest of your life?

Now, you may think the answer is obvious…you want the new, much better relationship. But you don't really know what this is yet, so you might want to wait a bit before you decide if you are truly willing to commit. For some people, this solution will be pure gold. For others, however, it may not make any difference— depending upon how open you are.

I have found that this approach is the best way out of this difficult problem—which most people never, ever solve—so I do encourage you do pay very close attention to this final step, because I believe it does hold the key to whether you succeed or fail in your quest to find lasting relief from your recurring irritability.

YOUR PRESENT AUTOMATIC RELATIONSHIP

As I pointed out in Step 2 of your master plan, your present relationship to feeling irritated (angry), once this occurs for you, can be described as looking for ways to suppress your irritability, hide the fact that you are feeling irritated, or express your feelings by letting others around you know how irritated they have made you feel.

I also explained that your present automatic relationship is built upon the presupposition that you are **justified** in feeling irritable, and that therefore the underlying thoughts, assumptions, and perceptions which are creating your feeling state **are accurate and correct**.

In other words, your present relationship to becoming angry and feeling irritated is to automatically assume that you have very good grounds for feeling irritated, and that the only issue remaining is to decide whether to suppress or express how you feel.

This is actually the crux of your problem. It is also, quite paradoxically, the door to achieving life-long irritability relief.

You see, the major reason why you continue to get irritated is not just that your body has become programmed to automatically think and behave in very specific ways that cause you to feel angry.

It is also because you automatically believe that your internal thoughts, beliefs, assumptions, perceptions, behaviors—and yes even your precious feelings—are actually valid, true, and completely justified!

This is your present, automatic relationship to feeling irritated. As I also pointed out in Step 2, this is the very same thing that people who commit road rage do, or that people who repeatedly verbally or physically abuse other people do.

It's the same fundamental relationship to feeling angry. So if you want to stop feeling irritated, you are going to have to do something different. You are going to have to create a different type of relationship to feeling irritated, each and every time this internal feeling starts to occur for you.

And this can't be just any type of relationship. It has to be a particular type of relationship—one that has the power to overcome the weakness of your automatic relationship and thereby set you free from having to suffer with continued anger and irritability.

The key to knowing what type of relationship to create, in order to get the relief you desire, is to understand that your present relationship is what's keeping your problem in place. It's also been the major barrier to you solving this problem on your own—up until now.

The primary aspect of your present relationship to feeling irritated—the one that is causing all your misery—is that it causes you to assume that each of your anger-producing thought patterns, and each of your anger-producing action patterns, which automatically gets triggered within you, really is true! In reality, however, much of the time—they are not!

This is why I told you, in Step 2, that when you stay with your automatic way of relating to your irritability, it will rarely occur to you that you may not actually have good grounds for feeling irritated, since your standard way of relating is to automatically assume just the opposite.

Thus, if you want to get free from your recurring irritability problem, *you are going to have to critically examine the specific thoughts and behaviors which are causing your angry feelings to occur, with a serious intention to try to discover where they might not be true.* Perhaps they are only partly true. Or maybe they are partly mistaken. Or in some cases, they may be totally false.

Either way, the new type of relationship you are going to need to create is one where you actively **attempt to disprove** your automatic thoughts, perceptions, feelings, etc. with the goal of trying to pinpoint exactly where they might be false—instead of automatically assuming that they are true.

GET GOOD AT THIS ONE SKILL AND YOUR LIFE WILL CHANGE—DRAMATICALLY!

This is the "secret sauce" I was referring to in Step 2 to knowing how to make your irritability lessen or quickly disappear. It's all about the type of relationship you choose to have towards your feelings of irritability and anger, including the thoughts, beliefs, perceptions, etc. that create them.

If you get very good at this one critically important skill—learning how to actively seek to disprove your automatic thoughts, feelings, and habitual behavior tendencies—your life will change dramatically. Not only will this one very important skill help you to rapidly decrease (or in some cases completely eliminate) your feelings of irritability whenever they occur, but it will also help you to deal with many other emotions and many other non-emotional problems in your life as well.

And fortunately for you—because you purchased and read this guide—you not only have an excellent master plan for finally solving your long-standing irritability problem, but you also have the golden key to help you do this successfully.

This **golden key**—which you now hold in your hand, and which many other people have no idea about—is that you now know exactly which specific thoughts and which specific behaviors are likely to be untrue!

YOUR ANGER INDEX CARD IS WORTH GOLD!

Your golden key to ultimately solving your irritability problem is the **Anger Index Card** we built together in Step 4 of your master plan.

Unlike most people alive today, you now know exactly what specific thought patterns and what specific action patterns are causing your anger/irritability to occur.

All you have to do now is look at each of the statements on your Anger Index Card and find out which of these (sometimes it will be all of them) are not really true!

It's actually like shooting wooden ducks on a pond, in that your targets are sitting right there in clear view, immobile in front of you, and all you have to do is aim straight and pull the trigger.

However, in real life, "shooting down" the specific thought patterns and action patterns which are causing you to feel angry, and which are sitting right in front of you on your Anger Index Card, is not always easy for people to do. At least it may be difficult initially.

There are two basic reasons for this:

1. You haven't spent very much time practicing the art of discovering that your automatic thoughts, feelings, and behavior tendencies aren't really true.

2. You are probably going to **actively resist** this exercise...because deep down inside, you really do believe that the way you see things,

think about things, and feel about things really is correct.

The only thing is...much of the time they are not! Much of the time, your feelings of irritation are not really justified. Not even close, to be brutally honest with you.

You already know this to be true because little things that irritate you don't really bother most other people. This tells you that you have to be blowing things way out of proportion. Unless you believe that most other people are dunces and you are one of the few truly smart people on the planet (which would be an excellent example of a thought you might believe in that's not really true).

You see, many of the automatic thoughts and perceptions we have turn out to be untrue when they are closely and critically examined. This was a regular source of enjoyment for the ancient Greek philosopher Socrates, who delighted in taking some of the brightest and wisest thinkers in Athens and showing them that most of what they believed to be absolutely true was pure B.S. when they were forced to examine each idea more closely.

Think about your own life for a moment. How many times have you gotten angry or irritated because you thought someone did something for a particular reason, only to find out later on that they had a completely different (and much more innocent) motive?

How many times have you judged someone's thoughts or behaviors as being "bad" or "wrong" when in actuality they were not? They only differed from what you believe or what you think is the best way to do things.

You No Longer Have To Rely Upon Luck To Find Out You Were Wrong

The good news is you no longer have to wait for good luck or good fortune to discover that something you assumed to be true several weeks ago actually turned out to be false.

You now can take immediate control of your own thought processes, and determine for yourself which ones are true and which ones are not.

You now have your Anger Index Card, so the moment you begin to feel irritated (or as close to that moment as possible) you can now be your own Socrates, or your own personal B.S. detector, and figure out for yourself where your automatic assumptions may be steering you wrong.

Once again, getting very good at this skill takes some work and lots of practice. It also doesn't happen overnight.

But the more you try it, and the more you practice examining the previously hidden internal sources of your anger, the better you will become at honing this skill, and the more you will start to see your feelings of anger and irritation quickly melt away...right before your eyes.

Also, the more you practice with your Anger Index Card, eventually the knowledge contained on this card will become second nature for you. When this happens, you'll be able to figure out, instantly, exactly why you got angry or felt irritated, without ever having to glance at your index card again.

CONCLUSION

I want to thank you and congratulate you for taking the time to read all the way through this self-help guide.

You now have the game plan (your 5-step master plan) and the golden key (your Anger Index Card) to finally take control of your irritability problem and end it once and for all.

It's one thing to tell someone to stop getting so upset over little things that really shouldn't bother them.

It's quite another, as I'm sure you'll agree, to show someone exactly how to do this. And hopefully, this is what I've been able to do for you in this guide.

Good luck with your ongoing efforts to stop being irritable, and if this guide does help you accomplish this goal, please let me know by emailing me your success story at docorman@gmail.com.

To your health, happiness, and success,

Doc Orman, M.D.

P.S. If you liked this book, I am developing an international community of like-minded people who are interested in achieving higher levels of stress reduction than stress management can provide.

I am building this community through my Stress Mastery Academy, and you are welcome to join us if you'd like. The cost is a one-time fee of less than $10, and this includes an excellent advanced training course on how to master stress, along with a subscription to our 52-week email newsletter.

You can find out more about how to join this Academy by going to **www.stressmasteryacademy.com** and downloading the free special report featured there.

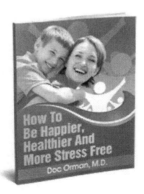

At the end of this report, you'll learn all about the Academy and the advanced training course you'll receive when you join.

OTHER BOOKS BY DOC ORMAN

Stress Relief Wisdom: Ten Key Distinctions For A Stress Free Life

The Choice Of Paradox: How "Opposite Thinking" Can Improve Your Life And Reduce Your Stres

The Ultimate Method For Dealing With Stress: How To Eliminate Anxiety, Irritability And Other Types Of Stress Without Having To Use Drugs, Relaxation Exercises Or Stress Management Techniques

The Art Of True Forgiveness: How To Forgive Anyone For Anything, Anytime You Want

Stop Negative Thinking: How To Stop Worrying, Relieve Stress, and Become a Happy Person Again

The Test Anxiety Cure: How To Overcome Exam Anxiety, Fear and Self Defeating Habits

The 14 Day Stress Cure: A New Approach For Dealing With Stress That Can Change Your Life

How To Have A Stress Free Wedding...And Live Happily Ever After

Sleep Well Again: How To Fall Asleep Fast, Stay Asleep Longer, And Get Better Sleep Like You Did In The Past

ABOUT THE AUTHOR

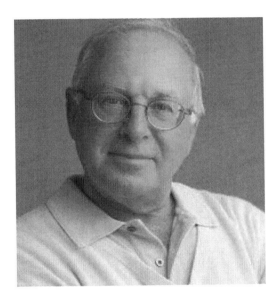

MORT (Doc) ORMAN, M.D. is an Internal Medicine physician, author, stress coach, and founder of the Stress Mastery Academy. He has been teaching people how to eliminate stress, without managing it, for more than 30 years. He has also conducted seminars and workshops on reducing stress for doctors, nurses, veterinarians, business executives, students, the clergy, and even the F.B.I.

Dr. Orman's award-winning book, The 14 Day Stress Cure (1991), is still one of the most helpful and innovative books on the subject of stress ever written. Dr. Orman and his wife, Christina, a veterinarian, live in Maryland.

43990372R00048

Made in the USA
San Bernardino, CA
04 January 2017